MEMORY

The enemy of memory creeps nearer and the mists thicken

for a while, then part again and roll away and sunshine gleams.

The joy is like a long forgotten thing of love returned;

But always the enemy is stalking and the fog not far away;

But if it never hides me from all time and memories;

Then I can live my life as I have always done;

My reason is still with me, only my memory is challenged,

And the enemy is held at bay.

Sadly, he will be with me always, but for now is still and held in check;

And I can live my life as always and laugh and think and be myself,

And full of joy and gratitude again;

And the cup of life still brims and laughter ripples and fond old memories

will never fade away.

David Barnato

South Africa 2014

This book is dedicated to my dearest wife Julian.

INTRODUCTION

It was when I was ordering a book on line from Amazon, that my memory went blank and I couldn't remember the name of the street where I lived. After fiddling around with my laptop I then couldn't recognize the icons on the screen. An absolute feeling of panic gripped me. It was as if a curtain of mist had descended like the end of a stage show. Then the curtain lifted for the players to take their congratulations .After a few moments my memory returned and I remembered my address, and the icons, but it was one of the most frightening experiences of my life, a bit like drowning in a sea of fog. I had previously experienced slight 'blank spots' but nothing like this. However, it finally propelled me to seek a medical opinion and so I went off yet again after several years, to see the quack.

As I drove I was probably in denial, but I thought that a few pills would put matters right. However, after listening to my symptoms of forgetting names and faces, cognitive difficulties, the blank spots and other problems, the doctor stated quite unequivocally that I was suffering from dementia and that there was no cure. He explained that there were some medications that might offer some respite, but in his opinion they were not very effective, had side effects and the cost was high. Rocked, as if by an earthquake, I struggled to accept this new and terrifying future. What exactly was dementia? I remembered people in my family had had, 'senile dementia.' They seemed to be 'old and crazy', but I didn't feel old, although I certainly wasn't young any more. It didn't seem possible that this could be happening to me.

Upon returning home and searching the internet my fear grew as I learned that dementia in itself is not a disease, but rather the symptom of something much worse to come and that from my particular symptoms, there was an 80% chance that this was Alzheimer's disease. I remembered how over almost twenty years the memory problems had grown worse. Forgetting where I had parked the car and not doing some of the things that I should have done, struggling with the internet, or balancing my cheque book and now the 'blank spots'.

My face in my hands, I sat and considered the horrifying future that lay ahead. The descent into total short term memory loss, and a life of constantly struggling to understand. To suffer a confused and frightening existence. The almost certain powerlessness and dependence on others and ultimately a death without dignity as the damaged brain eventually failed to send the simple message to the lungs to breathe! For me, who had had such a wonderful and full life, blessed in so many ways it was a truly shocking experience. I had travelled widely, run businesses, some successful and some not, but what a glorious time I had had. Even in retirement I had found a new career as a writer, or as some might say a 'scribler'.

It is not surprising that depression took over and for a while I wallowed in self pity and desperation. Then I remembered how in the past I had overcome depression without drugs and my usual optimistic nature re-asserted itself and after all, like that old song said; "There's got to be a little rain sometime."

 This book is about my experiences for over twenty years with memory loss,   which was finally recognized as dementia. It is this and the possibility of Alzheimer disease, that at age seventy two   I am now fighting with considerable success and living my life fully and joyfully.

It was a big shock to be told that I had dementia, but the decision to fight came quickly. Although some damage has been done and I have difficulty recognizing names and faces and I sometimes struggle for the odd word, and have other problems, I have been able to write this book and to almost arrest my dementia. How this happened is what this book is all about and the method used can be used by any sufferer, particularly those in the early stages and even as a way for young people to look after their brain, as they should look after their heart, and avoid dementia and Alzheimer's in later life. Sometimes the disease is inherited, rather than 'caused`, but the advance can be delayed until a much later stage. Those in latter stage Alzheimer's can also dramatically improve the quality of their lives, particularly if they have good care givers, and indeed this book has been written with both early stage dementia patients and care givers in mind. Part one is written for dementia sufferers like myself. It explains how it feels to have dementia and what one can do about it. The second part is advice for caregivers and those dementia sufferers who can still understand and still read. What most people don't realize is that dementia and Alzheimer's doesn't remove a person's intelligence, but rather the ability to access and use intelligence, thus many patients with dementia will be able to understand their illness and the procedures that help minimize dementia and Alzheimer's. The book is not intended to be a great and detailed treatise, that can be found elsewhere. It is a simple way to fight dementia and to provide simple information and advice for new caregivers. The advice given to those diagnosed with dementia is not difficult to follow and the small amount of self discipline called for will be rewarded many times over by better health and a better memory.

I am not a medical doctor and so you must take professional advice before following the ideas made here. They have certainly helped me to stop the deterioration that was taking place. I hope with all my heart that they will work for you.

PART ONE

I FORGET WHAT I FORGOT

CHAPTER ONE

WHAT IT FEELS LIKE TO LEARN THAT ONE HAS DEMENTIA

Although my memory difficulties had crept up on me over an almost twenty year period, it was still a shock to be told that I had dementia. During the years of my dementia, I had visited doctors and had Alzheimer's tests several times about my poor memory, with good results. It was this perhaps that left me with a feeling of false security.

It was when I started experiencing blank spots that I became worried. Several times I had forgotten that I had already done errands that were scheduled. It was almost more than forgetting, there was just a blank where the memory of the event should have been. In addition, my memory of events had deteriorated and my memory for people and names had become considerably worse. My orientation was deteriorating and I experienced spatial difficulties which made me stumble or knock my head. Solving problems was also becoming more difficult, particularly in respect of using the computer. This presented quite a big challenge for me, as since retiring I had become a writer and published a couple of books on Amazon.

As I drove home from the doctors I felt my spirits quail. Almost numb with shock I tried to fathom just what this meant to me in real terms and being optimistic by nature, I decided to investigate what dementia was and how to fight it.

If I was worried at the beginning of my first day of my research, by the end of the day I was even more devastated. The possibility of Alzheimer's seemed very high, as I had all the symptoms. However, there was not yet any way of confirming the presence of Alzheimer's, although a blood test analysis would be available by the end of 2014.In addition, it was stated that there was no known cure for either Alzheimer's or dementia.

There were 70 million Alzheimer sufferers throughout the world I discovered, of which 5 million were in the United States and almost one million in the UK.

My feelings of despair returned. A slow, but inevitable road of increasing debilitations lay ahead. My individuality would go and I would lose my ability to run my own life and eventually lose completely control of my own existence. I thought of the people who would have little sympathy and probably despise me as I became foolish from the disease. In addition ,if illnesses associated with advancing Alzheimer's hadn't already killed me, Alzheimer's disease itself would do so, because the increasing damage to the brain would eventuality mean that the brain would stop even sending the necessary messages to the body to breathe.

At that moment in time I felt as if I was in a mist and in my mind what lay ahead as an inevitable and continuous thickening of the mist and ultimately a complete fog. The feeling of hopelessness was crushing, and it was as if a steel band was around my head and being tightened.

Then I felt myself come 'back on track' and work steadily to understand and meet the challenges and I felt my spirits soar .It was impossible for me to just let this happen. Surely there must be a cure? We had been sending men into space for many years. Our cell phones are now computers and cameras as well and every kid on every street corner of the world had one. To many, these 'phones' were almost an extension of their bodies. The internet had changed the world as much as the railways had, less than two hundred years before .With the advances in medical science, populations were living longer everywhere Surely there had to be a way to at least arrest Alzheimer's disease, even if the damage done couldn't be reversed. Sadly this was not the case I learned, there was nothing that main stream medical science could do, although there were some drugs that for some people were giving some comfort, but my own doctor had dismissed them as being of little medical value and very expensive. His only advice was a careful diet and to use the brain as much as possible to delay the advance of the disease. We looked at one another and I realized that there was nothing that he could offer me and in a way I felt that he had written me off and so I politely thanked him and left.

As I walked to my car I remember feeling so alone that it was almost unbearable, it was like being cast adrift in a small boat and being pulled towards a waterfall that lay ahead.

When I mentioned to a friend the other day that my dementia was actually a symptom of something worse and that there was an 80% chance of it being Alzheimer's he made a joke.

"The one good thing about Alzheimer's is that you get to meet new people every day."

I laughed, but I was a bit shocked and then when I reflected on it, I realized that in fact humour was an essential ingredient to fighting dementia and Alzheimer's.

As a young man I could drive 500 miles along the twisty winding roads of those days and remember every bend, every parking space and every 'greasy spoon' café where a cup of stewed English tea could be bought and something called 'coffee' which tasted more like mud and required lots of sugar to even be palatable. I could also remember the varying degrees of running fat in a bacon sandwich for each café on the route. Perhaps it is the boring sameness of the eateries on the British motorways today that makes me forget them and perhaps it is the dreariness of driving along the soulless routes that makes them unworthy of memory retention.

However, by the time that I was fifty I began to be aware of my deteriorating memory. I had parked my car, but I couldn't remember where! This was serious enough for me to visit Doctor Stephens our local GP who gave me a test for Alzheimer's disease, which I passed with flying colours yet again. "Don't worry old chap," He said cheerfully. " Failing memory is quite normal past fifty."

So I left the surgery a much happier man and unworried about my memory and unfortunately uninformed about how to look after my memory. My late wife and I were also mistaken about our physical health and continued to smoke, drink steadily and heavily, and to follow a very popular diet that certainly worked for weight, but was also undermining our health, and in my particular case, my memory in particular was I think in part being damaged by the diet and lifestyle.

Good health is the first step in maintaining both a healthy heart and a sound mind and memory, but our way of eating was a disaster. The diet was almost totally non carbohydrate, but one could eat butter, lots of fat, cream, and loads of eggs. In addition, as there were no carbohydrates in whisky, brandy and good French wine, we could really enjoy an epicurean lifestyle and live forever. The cigarettes of my wife and my smoky cigars were conveniently forgotten. We worked hard at our business and we also played hard.

Five years ago at age fifty nine my wife was dead and soon afterwards, my previously perfect health began to collapse. The many bodily pains were diagnosed as being caused by blocked arteries and an operation by that wonderful surgeon Andrew Murray of Cape Town to insert a 'stent' saved my life.

My bodily health quickly recovered and two years later when I married Julian my improved diet and regime of exercise and the abolition of alcohol and tobacco gave me a fresh start. I still had a lot of mysterious pains though and my memory was getting worse.

There is a great deal of information available on the internet and a large number of organizations helping Alzheimer and dementia sufferers. There is a lot of good advice and so I began to take Trimega, Omega three tablets and having heard that macadamia nuts also helped these were included in my new diet.

It is very difficult to tell if a particular medicine or food is helping with this problem, but my memory was still getting slowly but steadily worse. Then, I became ill with a stomach bug. This was the most virulent bug that I have ever suffered. My son in law who also lived with us went down on the same day. He was a normally healthy twenty six year old, but he was off and on unconscious for two days and ill for weeks. In my own case I ended up in Hospital on a drip.

There is no need to go into graphic detail and indeed to do so would certainly put the reader off his next meal, or even worse. Suffice to say that it involved being assisted to the loo about twenty five times a day for two weeks.

We were ill for about a month, but as a result of the illness there was in my case one huge benefit that revealed to me how dementia and thus Alzheimer's could be dramatically slowed down and even arrested.

CHAPTER TWO

GETTING ILL MADE ME BETTER

The doctor had warned me that the greatest danger was de-hydration, so I drank a lot of water. This was not difficult, as for the first week I ate almost nothing and very little on the second. Drinking lots of water was not a problem, as during this period I had a raging thirst. In fact I was only tempted to start eating sparingly when the cramps finally ended after two weeks.

The discomfort and pain had gone and my body was working normally, but I felt utterly drained and exhausted. A massive vitamin injection propelled me into recovery and after a month I felt wonderful and after resuming walking and swimming I felt ten years younger and in excellent health.

It was my wife Julian who explained that because of my loss of body fluids throughout the illness, my body had been purged of poisons and I had in fact had experienced a massive detox. It was whilst I was convalescing that I realized that the advance of my memory loss was considerably reduced.

In the months that followed I came to realize that there were many things that effected memory and many ways in which the young might prevent dementia and Alzheimer's in later life. For those like me, suffering from dementia and probably Alzheimer's the steps to be taken could at the very least slow down dementia and Alzheimer's, and possibly arrest it as well.

The 'detox' that my body had undergone gave me the first clue that memory loss, dementia and Alzheimer's were very much linked to not only bodily health, but mental and spiritual health as well. So a new regime began and almost by accident I heard about coconut oil. Apparently, a doctor in the US whose husband had Alzheimer's introduced him to coconut oil and in 37 days his illness had completely stopped advancing. There are now, after several years tens of thousands of people who testify that coconut oil has helped either them or their partners

. In the following months I felt fitter and younger and my memory was now almost stable. It was obvious to me that it was a combination of the various parts of the 'cure' that was the key. It was not enough to have a healthy body achieved by modest exercise and a carefully selected diet, it was essential to have a healthy mind and brain achieved by mental stimulus. But even these important steps were not the whole solution. A holistic approach was called for and the spirit also needed exercise, which called for 'prayer' and meditation.

SPIRITUAL HEALTH

To many, the concept of 'prayer' will be a difficult one to accept, but my experience of life has shown that even atheists believe that there must be something greater than oneself. Even if you do not believe in God, believe in the Universe, or even the ether if you prefer, but believe in something greater than yourself. The contact that will follow will be prayer. Almost everyone now believes in positive thinking. . Personally I pray to God himself.

Meditation is something that I have practiced for many years on an irregular basis and has given me insights into many things. The state of calmness achieved is quite wonderful and when linked to the physical, mental and spiritual, a healthy and happy life state can be reached.

Meditation is regarded by many people with great mystique. However, the deep states achieved by gurus etc., are not necessary, simple meditation is sufficient. The following method was taught to me by the Rosicrucians, whose Grand Master was the late Christian Barnard the heart transplant pioneer.

MEDITATION

A darkened room is best with a lit candle to focus on and ideally a mirror behind. The latter is not essential, but does enable one to 'look into oneself' and achieve a deeper meditative state.

Light an incense stick and play soothing classical music. Even better, buy a cd recorded for meditation. Tim Wheater the flautist who is my brother has produced a number of these for healing. [Tim Wheater .com]

Breathe deeply and hold your breath for a moment. Continue to slowly breathe in and out gently, deeply and rhythmically until you are completely relaxed. Then imagine that you are under a gentle shower and the water trickling down your body is washing away all worry and stress. It runs from your head and down over your body taking any stress with it.

Close your eyes and in your mind visualize a special place. It can be a valley, a mountain top, or even a building. This will be your special place that you will go to every time when meditating.

Imagine that you are walking towards your special place and when you reach it let your mind and imagination think of healing. Think of your memory, it is getting better. Just visualize.

If you suffer from depression think of the good things in your life. Perhaps they are small, but if you think about it, every single day there is something to be grateful for. Count your blessings and let the depression and worry flow out of your body. There will always be someone worse off than yourself, as there will also be someone better off than you. Just think of the good things. If you have bad things in your life ask God or the Great Spirit or the Universe to send you a solution. Then switch back to happiness.

You can spend as long as you like meditating, there is no ideal time, I usually meditate for about half an hour.

CHAPTER THREE

EXERCISE

Personally I have never been a great fan of strenuous exercise. I have not been to a gym since my schooldays and the horror of the tortures experienced there and the exhaustion from cross country running haunts me to this day! However, when I was young we walked a lot. Not just from necessity, but just for the joy, and swimming, provided the temperature was high enough was another pleasure. In fact when I was about twelve I even swam in the sea early every morning, it was not actually a pleasure but the result of a bet.

In those days we lived on the Isle of Wight, a small island off the south coast of England at a place called Gurnard. We were about two hundred yards from the beach. One day I was with my parents who were visiting friends. The conversation got round to our planned family holiday to Cornwall. In those distant civilized days children were generally seen and not heard, but somehow I became involved with the conversation and mentioned how little my holiday funds were. The lady of the house challenged me swim every day for three months; "If you can do it David you'll have won ten shillings."

This was an enormous sum in the early fifties and being a very enterprising boy I faithfully followed the terms of the bet and swam every morning. It was early summer, but those aware of the temperature of the English Channel will know that if a brass monkey were to enter the water, parts of its anatomy would fall off. However, I quite enjoyed the challenge and duly claimed my reward. The lady concerned was astounded when I told her that I had honoured the bet, but believed me and paid up. Many years later I learned that the currents in the sea where I swam were actually very dangerous, but I survived.

However, in my experience an hours walk a day is quite sufficient exercise to stay healthy. In fact I recently read on the net that one hour's walking per day will extend one's life by seven years. Personally I also swim forty lengths in my swimming pool when temperatures permit. I should however point out that my pool is very small, so this is not quite such an enormous achievement as it sounds. On rainy days I walk for fifteen minutes on my treadmill. But there is no doubt that exercise is a part of a healthy life style, for both mind and body, but it doesn't have to be boring or exhaustive, many people still dance into their eighties. For those unable to walk I would suggest talking to a professional about lifting weights or some other form of exercise that you can do. My own father was lifting simple weights until he died at eighty.

EXERCISE OF THE MIND

This is just as important for the memory as walking or other forms of exercise are for the body. When I was young before television became universal, we listened to the radio, played chess and other games and we read. We read a lot and it saddens me to see today how many people don't read at all and others only occasionally. Of course many people now read e books, particularly when travelling, but books are not the sacred things that they once were. When I was a young man we talked a lot about authors and their books. It was a very common topic and most people were reading something specific and it was routine to ask one's fiends what they were currently reading.

Books play an enormous role in helping the elderly to delay the progress of Alzheimer's and for the young this healthy exercise of the mind can, if combined with healthy living, delay the onset of memory loss and perhaps prevent dementia and Alzheimer's.

Playing chess, drafts, crosswords, learning a language and conversation also exercise the mind and so does writing creatively and painting. There is also some benefit to be gained from television documentaries, films and even some soaps. However, it is not healthy for the mind to rely exclusively on the passive watching of television for long periods. As with everything in life, balance is essential and there is great benefit to be had from social networking, but don't forget the other meaningful ways that the mind can be exercised. Also, social contact with friends and family should be continued as much as possible.

Like the physical exercise part of life, mental exercise doesn't have to be boring. Just be aware that you need to stimulate your mind.

MUSIC

Music plays a big part in all our lives and research shows that babies and young children exposed to gentle classical music perform better academically than others. Certainly in the case of Alzheimer patients at all stages, music calms; particularly so in the case of those in the latter stages of Alzheimer disease. In the past they were often treated as beyond contact, almost like vegetables. Many of us have visited old peoples' homes, and been saddened by the slumped, and unconscious looking figures in wheelchairs, regarded as beyond hope. However, we now know that with love, patience and knowledge these patients can often be reached and in fact they are often only sleeping and not in vegetative comas. The procedure is to stroke the patient's face as a mother would a child and play music from the era when the patient was young. Then talk to the patient gently. There is a remarkable video of this process actually happening. In it the elderly lady care giver sings a hymn to the even older patient and the lady begins to respond and eventually they sing the hymn together. It is quite beautiful to watch and demonstrates so well how music and love can heal.

Music really does play an important part in healing and preventing illness.

DIET

There is very definitely a correlation between what we eat and our memory. However, before listing the foods that are believed to positively help memory let me say that an occasional lapse into the 'bad foods' will happen .It's not ideal, but probably not a 'train smash`, so just resume healthy eating and be determined that lapses will only be occasional and don't stress. Stress is perhaps a major cause of dementia and Alzheimer's.

The first ' good food' is not really a food, but in my experience has helped me tremendously in every way, and by boosting my health has I am sure helped me to stop memory deterioration. This amazing thing is WATER. It is ironic that the availability of good water has increased globally, but I suspect that the drinking of water on its own has decreased. Water used to make rooibos tea, or green tea is water well drunk, but the water in fizzy drinks is almost completely wasted. Water on its own is truly God's gift and I start the day with a full glass and I make sure that I drink about two liters of water per day. On the rare occasions when I experience pain or discomfort I drink a glass of water and the pain is 'washed away.' No doubt part of this particular success comes from positive thinking, but I am utterly convinced of the efficacy of water, but I try to control the amount drunk in the evening to reduce the need to urinate overnight.

So water is top of my food list. However, the very first step in the 'Barnato Plan to health' is to DETOX your body using one of the many herbal methods, but do please speak to your doctor before you start. A detox is so important to rid the body of toxins, and I feel that it was the accidental key to my success in dramatically slowing down my dementia. When I first became aware of this I remembered almost sixty years ago, when I was working on a farm in Spain. The old English gentleman who owned the farm told me about his father, who had been a medical doctor. Of course he would have been practicing in young Queen Victoria's reign, but the Victorians were very clever people! Doctor Williams believed totally in the efficacy of an annual purge. This would be a combination of fasting and taking a mild laxative and of course drinking lots and lots of water. As my elderly friend was in his nineties and very fit and compos mentis when he told me about this, I think it reasonable to suppose that it is a good idea. However, talk to your doctor before commencing this 'cure`!

Next come fruit and vegetables, particularly the ones in the list. Some of the fruits are expensive but less so in season. If however budget is a constraint, just focus on the fruit that is cheap in your country. In South Africa where I live, bananas are almost always cheap, but other fruits are only affordable in season. So the choice depends on where you live and your budget.

Some fish such as pilchards and salmon are rich in omegas and it is generally believed, definitely help with the memory, others less so. Meat should be eaten moderately and red meat with fat avoided if possible. So chicken and ostrich meat are acceptable and both lend themselves to a vast range of dishes.

All cakes, biscuits, and sweets and processed foods should be avoided, or eaten very occasionally as treats, because excessive sugar and salt is bad for the brain. Pure chocolate in moderation can be eaten and my wife and I drink a cup of cocoa with cinnamon and a teaspoonful of honey first thing in the morning [after a glass of water] and last thing at night. This ritual began after a friend of ours had been told to do so and was convinced of the health benefits. We have no evidence of these, but by golly it tastes good! Bread should be whole meal and low GI., and eaten sparingly. Pasta and rice are also good foods, especially brown rice, but they are not as positively beneficial as the foods in the list.

A study of two groups of mice over nine months showed interesting results. Those fed on a high calorie and high carbohydrate diet all had plaques on the brain similar to those in humans that cause dementia and Alzheimer's. Those fed on a normal rodent diet had none. Of course mice aren't people, but the tests do seem to confirm very specifically that diet is a critical factor in memory loss and dementia. Scientists believe that the low carbohydrate and low calorie diet may have unleashed a chemical chain reaction that stopped the plaque development and thus stopped damage to the brain, experienced by dementia and Alzheimer patients. The question of correct weight for one's size also seems to be relevant to the advance of dementia and Alzheimer's.

Another factor in dealing with dementia and Alzheimer's is vitamin intake. A study carried out over 5 years of 4740 participants aged 65 and over, found that those on vitamins C and A supplements reduced their risk of Alzheimer's by 64%.

Magnesium is good for brain functioning and vitamin E is also believed to specifically good for the brain and thus the memory.

Alcohol should be very limited or avoided. A glass of red wine per day is regarded by many as being beneficial, but in my experience it is easier to abstain from alcohol than reduce it, but this is a personal choice.

In my experience it is not difficult to stop drinking. Before I did so, I thought that it would be very difficult, as I couldn't imagine life without a drink at five o'clock but in fact the only thing that I found a problem was the decision to stop. However, this will not be the case with everyone. If drinking is a problem to you then you must seek professional advice. The one almost certainty is that excessive alcohol destroys brain cells as well as damages the liver etc.

SMOKING

Unlike most boys I did not start smoking until I was eighteen and then only to impress a girl. I stopped smoking cigarettes ten years later, but then ten years after that I commenced smoking cigars. In those days we were told that nicotine was the culprit and cigars and pipe tobacco not harmful if we didn't inhale.

However, my heart surgeon absolutely assured me that the smoke from my cigars had contributed heavily towards my blocked arteries and almost killed me. As there can be no doubt that smoking is not beneficial and is almost certainly very harmful, it should be avoided by the young to stay healthy and the old to stay alive! There is little doubt that smoking is bad for the health and therefore bad for the memory.

To stop smoking is for most people very difficult. In fact I personally know people who were able after a struggle to give up hard drugs but couldn't stop smoking cigarettes.

In my own case it was harder to stop smoking cigarettes all those years ago but very easy to give up the cigars more recently. In both cases though, the difficult part is the decision. Only the decision!

To stop smoking cigarettes first make the decision. Then compose a mantra to repeat to yourself every time you crave a cigarette. An example might be; "If I smoke a cigarette again I will be sick."

Each time you think of a cigarette take a stick of chewing gum instead. Until you have really given up reduce your social activities if possible, or try and limit your circle to non smokers. Other people who smoke will be your greatest difficulty. If you struggle to give up try the artificial cigarettes, they do seem to work for some people.

SLEEP

Personally, I have sleeping difficulties and so I take a sleeping pill. Health conscious people would I am sure say that sleeping pills are harmful, but it is a personal decision. However, at least seven hours sleep per night is essential to almost everyone. Some people need eight, but very few need less and much illness is caused by sleep starvation. From research and tests it is almost certain that lack of sleep damages the brain and thus the memory.

Although it is possible to survive on less sleep, over a long period damage will be done. If you have to get up early to let the dog out, go to bed early, or if possible take a nap in the

15

afternoon. However, although beneficial, I find that sleep in the afternoon should be limited to avoid insomnia at night.

THE FOODS FOR MEMORY

Apart from omega 3 and 6 fatty acid tablets and plenty of water there are many foods that aid the memory. However, out of the list that follows there are six foods that are believed to positively aid memory. The five foods are COCONUT OIL, SPINACH, STRAWBERRIES, BLUEBERRIES, MACADAMIA NUTS AND DE-FATTED SOY FLOUR.

There are now a great number of people who claim enormous benefit from coconut oil in particular and I also now include this as part of my diet. When I first tried the two teaspoons recommended three times a day as a food supplement, I found that it made me feel very nauseous and rather ill. However, Dr. Mary Newport who wrote 'Alzheimer's Disease: What If There Were a Cure?' advised a number of ways that coconut oil could be taken and the oily taste masked.

In the book she tells the story of how in 2008 she introduced coconut oil to her husband Steve who was suffering from Alzheimer's and she claims how in only 37 days his Alzheimer's was reversed.

Although I made great strides in slowing the advance of dementia before taking the coconut oil, I am convinced that the almost halting of the advance came from this final step.

To make it more palatable I mix some coconut oil with my Scottish style porridge known as 'Jungle Oats' by many, for breakfast and I also add some yoghurt. In addition I make 'magic chocolates.' To make these I melt three tablespoons of coconut oil in the microwave for thirty seconds. Then I mix in the same quantity of cocoa, the same of honey and a little glucose with a little boiling water. Then four desert spoons of milk, a table spoon of crushed macadamia nuts and finally a tablespoon of sugar. Mix thoroughly and pour into ice cube containers and freeze for about an hour. Then store in the fridge. I eat two or three chocolates a day after lunch and dinner and the number created from the above mix lasts for about one week.

The following is a long list of positive foods, so there is plenty of choice. Good quality food supports optimal brain function and boosts memory by providing essential nutrients. Also, antioxidant rich foods help improve the surge of oxygen through the brain as well as the body, thus aiding the memory.

THE THIRTY NINE GREAT FOODS

Coconut oil, alfalfa sprouts, beets, red bell peppers, onions, sweet potatoes, raspberries, plums, cabbage ,lettuce, spinach, kiwi fruits, cinnamon, honey, avocados, oranges, red grapes, cherries, red apples, kale, brussel- sprouts, red tomatoes, blueberries, blackberries, macadamia nuts, cranberries, strawberries, broccoli, green tea, rooibos tea, salmon, sardines, halibut, herring, tuna, mackerel, muesli. In addition some people claim most strongly that de-fatted soya flour made into breads or cakes are very beneficial.

It is noticeable that the list includes some fish but no meat. This does not mean that a healthy diet can't include some meat, but rather that meat is not an aid to memory. Meats that can be eaten are chicken and ostrich. Red meats should be eaten very occasionally and fatty meat excluded. If your religion permits it, lean pork can be eaten in moderation, but not the crackling.

We are what we eat, so care is needed to not only retain the memory and to keep the heart healthy, but also to retain good health generally Some people will stick religiously to this list, but personally I see no harm in the occasional piece of cake or juicy tea bone steak. The word of course is 'occasional `, but like all things in life, balance is important. However, at least one of the 'good foods' should be eaten every day and ideally each meal should include one good food. Bread, eggs, and other additional foods should be eaten sparingly. Sugar and extra salt should be avoided if possible. Personally, I am also very convinced of the benefits of honey and yogurt, but I have found no evidence that they are positively helpful to memory.

SUPPLEMENTS THAT SOME PEOPLE CLAIM HELP COMBAT ALZHEIMER'S

In her book 'Awakening From Alzheimer's' ,Peggy Sarlin lists nine possible ways to combat Alzheimer's, including coconut oil. There are examples in the book of many people who have benefited from the other ideas and supplements. However, at the present time there does not seem to be any recognition of the effectiveness of these remedies from mainstream science. That does not of course mean that they don't work and indeed coconut oil has helped myself and many thousands of others.

Apart from Omega 3 and 6 one should take vitamin supplements, but do discuss this with your doctor.

DEPRESSION

Depression is a huge problem for millions of people and I have certainly suffered from it in my life. In fact wanting to help others with the problem, I once joined 'The Samaritans,' a voluntary organization dedicated to helping people contemplating suicide. It was a very interesting experience and I was sadly aware of the quiet desperation that many people live with. Although I did advise and I think help a lot of people, in the end I just had to give up, because my work was exacerbating my own depression. I really do admire Samaritan volunteers who are able to selflessly help others, month after month and year after year.

However, eventually over a period of years I came to realize through meditation, the enormous number of blessings in my life and whenever my thoughts veered towards sadness and self- pity I was able to steer them back again to gratitude. Thankfully, I have retained this ability and by self- discipline I don't allow depression to stay in my thinking. It is not easy, but I think that anyone and everyone can reduce their depression, although I accept that for many it is very difficult and medication may have to be used. Even 'reactive depression', which is caused by actual bad experiences such as illness or death of a loved one, can often be controlled. A level of sadness for such an event is perfectly normal, but by thinking about the good things about the person, or the experience one's thinking can become more positive and depression controlled. Of course some bad things in life happen without the sufferer doing anything. In the case of Alzheimer's the only answer is to fight the disease and just not allow depression to take over. For those of a religious disposition the biblical 'Put your trust in the Lord and be still'; may be the only answer.

In my own case most depression was not caused by actual events, but just happened. Medication may be the only answer for many people, but positive thinking is best!

So the 'Barnato Health Plan' is a holistic approach of health of body, mind and spirit. The exercise of all three is essential to health. If young people adopt this plan there will be a higher chance that their life will be long, healthy and happy.

For those, like myself in the early stages of dementia the plan will at the very least slow down the deterioration towards Alzheimer's or whichever other disease you are suffering from. In my own case deterioration has almost stopped. Of course there is no known way to 'go back` and restore the damage to the brain. So I still have difficulty remembering names and faces. Sometimes I still forget words that I should remember and dealing with the complexities of my computer remains a challenge. However, there are grandchildren growing up who will soon be able to help me with that problem! Also, my co-ordination is slightly damaged and so I am more prone to bang my head or trip and stumble.

In some other ways I am tempted to say that my memory and cognitive abilities are marginally better. However, I suspect that is because I feel so good in my healthy, happy lifestyle. But I do know that there is almost no further deterioration taking place. Although one must be humble, they say that Alzheimer's is like a clock that loses a second a day, you don't notice it until you lose minutes. The answer I feel is to enjoy every day and try to remember the blessings that happen on even the bleakest day.

Perhaps being a writer is helping in my fight, certainly my ability, modest as it is, remains the same, apart from the occasional struggle to remember a word. However, with a little mental effort the word usually pops into my mind. Occasionally I have to use the Thesaurus, but then I have always used the Thesaurus to source extra words, as I have always used a diary to remember appointments etc.

For those in the early stages of dementia there is every hope that with attention to health your dementia can be reversed or at least slowed down and your life continue, fruitfully and happily as mine has done. For those in latter stages the same should apply, but of course the damage already done will be greater and as what is lost in the brain cannot be recovered, there will be greater difficulty in managing both memory and tasks. However, life can still go on for many without a caregiver, in the same way as many disabled people manage on their own with very severe difficulties such as blindness. Of course if you are fortunate enough to have a loving caregiver, then you will be blessed indeed.

For those people in one of the early stages of dementia, what I propose, will be understood and if practiced, your life can be much more positive.

Patients in the latter stages of Alzheime'rs may not be able to understand my health proposals. For those people, it is their caregivers who hopefully will get some benefit from this book and apply some of the ideas to your patients. Many caregivers already know all of these and more!

When one is diagnosed with dementia one contemplates a lot. My feeling is that my own dementia is almost permanently arrested and it is certainly contained for the time being. However, it may be that at a latter stage it will advance again, I pray not, but I accept that it could.

Because of this I have written a number of short notes for my wife Julian. These are advice notes following some personal experience, but mainly gleaned from research. Most of that research has been obtained from books and the internet, but I have also met and talked with dementia sufferers and their caregivers and the caregivers of Alzheimer's patients. These insights will be not only of interest to others, but I think some will be very useful.

May you all be blessed as I have been.

PART TWO

LETTERS TO MY WIFE JULIAN, IF MY DEMENTIA SHOULD GET WORSE

My Dear Julian,

You will I know, read these 'letters', not only if my condition worsens, but as a matter of interest and information . We both hope and expect that my condition will get no worse, but just in case I have written advice not only about dementia, but Alzheimer's as well. You are a remarkable woman and know that should I get worse I can put my trust in both yourself and God.

Love, David.

FIRST LETTER TO JULIAN

My Dear, at present the damage caused by dementia is limited and with planning and organization I am able to function very well indeed. My memory has flaws, but I have learned how to accept these and also how to recall words that I need. With the advice and help of others the cognitive damage is also under control.

The result is that our daily life continues very happily and you don't at present need help in looking after me .In the mornings I write and in the afternoons I read. In the evenings we watch a little television, listen to music or make social visits. As my condition is now stable and there has been very little deterioration in the past twelve months we have every expectation that there will be very little further deterioration. As a result we have not discussed who will help you should I become 'non compos mentis', but my advice is that whilst I remain at home with you, a helper be brought in for day care, leaving you to deal with me at night. This would enable you to have some breaks during the day from the very demanding responsibilities of looking after a patient in the middle, or late stages of dementia or Alzheimer's. However, should I get worse the next step will be into middle dementia. This is an extension of the difficulties already experienced in the early stages and I understand one can remain at this stage for many years, but let us remain optimistic and that I will remain in the early stages of dementia. This should enable me to stay at home with you, provided that you have some help.

Quite apart from the dementia challenge there is also the usual question of ageing and if I become feeble in my eighties it is essential that you get support if you can, to enable you to take a break away when possible. This is a sincere wish on my part to enable you to continue for what could be a number of years. Also, if possible you should use day care facilities where I could be left for a few hours a day for as long as practicable.

It will be very difficult for you to look after me at home in the latter stages of Alzheimer's, if God forbid I reach that stage! You must feel no guilt if the day comes when coping becomes dreadful, or even impossible. Investigate care homes and find one suitable and affordable. One of the things to be wary of apparently, is if the place smells of urine! Also, I have read that the number of caregivers per patient should be at least nine during the day and five at night .It is also as you know, very important that the care home practices the 'non confrontational' method of dealing with Alzheimer's victims. Many nurses are still unaware that it is not kind to tell a patient who wants to visit their mother, that she has been dead for forty years. Not only is the 'truth' often very disturbing for the patient, but also my lead to disturbed behavior which will put more stress on the caregiver. Also, 'wanting to go home' can mean many things and often not the last home, so the difficulty is best dealt with by diverting the patient's attention to a happy older memory.

Of course affordability may be an issue, so you must use your own discretion. Above all don't feel guilt, in fact I have read that it is a kindness to most people in the latter stages of Alzheimer's to use a care home because of the number of caregivers and medical facilities.

However, please do visit me at least once a week. You now know from our research, that although a patient may look 'vegetative', the real ' me` will still be inside. I may be sleeping but you may reach me by caressing my face as a mother would a child and playing some of the beautiful music that I like. There are so many wonderful pieces, but my favorite you will know is from Madame Butterfly, it is very sad, but I love it so!

If things reach the point where I am in care you will feel lonely. You have your deep religious faith and I know that that and the love of your children will sustain you. Please be happy in every way that you can. At least I leave you a vast library of books.

When I am finally gone, you know that I will be with my Redeemer, so don't feel sad for me, sing a song or a hymn at my funeral and bury me under a tree, if a space is available, in Paarl.

These things said, know that I intend to live my life to the full until the end. I expect to live a full and healthy life for many years yet. Indeed you will remember that I once met an Indian Guru who made a prophecy that I would live to be ninety two and die in my own bed. I expect to live the prophecy!

David

SECOND LETTER TO JULIAN

WHAT IS DEMENTIA?

This letter is not so much for you Julian as you already know so much about it, but other readers may like to know the facts. However, you will remember that although I had had many Alzheimer tests over the years which I 'passed`. When finally, I was definitely diagnosed as suffering from dementia, I was to say the least dismayed. I felt as if my long life was going to end quickly, or even worse my sanity would gradually disappear as the destruction of the brain continued until I was completely lost. If only I had known those things many years before dementia had commenced and been informed how to change my life style and diet.

At the time of my definite diagnosis, my dementia took the form of not only forgetting things, but 'blank spots' as well. It was as if a mist of forgetfulness would descend from time to time and I sometimes had no recollection of doing things. These were not bad things that I had done, just mundane shopping things or visits to the bank., but the point was that I had forgotten them. All in all it was a very dispiriting experience, and I felt a great dread of the future, but I immersed myself in research to find out what was happening to me. The good news is that at the time of writing this book I have had no more 'blank spots` and my memory loss has stabilized.

So, mainly for the benefit of those who have been recently diagnosed with dementia and also for potential caregivers, here is a simple explanation of dementia. It is not intended to be an exhaustive work on the subject. Much more detailed and technical information is available on line. This is just a simple guide.

Dementia is the symptom of the gradual loss of brain function because of brain damage caused by Alzheimer disease in 80% of patients; or Parkinsons, Multiple Sclerosis, Pick Disease, Progressive Supranclear Palsy, small strokes, diabetes, perhaps depression or brain injury in most of the others. There is currently no known cure for either dementia or Alzheimer's disease, but they can be slowed down dramatically in many cases.

The possible causes of these conditions are chronic alcohol abuse damaging the brain; brain tumors, brain injury, changes in blood sugar, or the use of certain medicines, including some anti cholesterol drugs and perhaps stress and smoking. Also, vitamin deficiency ,incorrect diet and a diet with excessive calories and carbohydrates. In addition, if you have a family history of dementia, there will be a possibility of the disease developing, which despite all the good steps that you take in early life may still develop. However, evidence suggests that the more sensibly that you live, the longer you will delay the onset of dementia and Alzheimer's. Also, bear in mind that it is not automatic that you will develop Alzheimer's just because there is a family history.

The symptoms of dementia are a gradual reduction in memory, often including 'blank spots', difficulties with language, perception and thinking and judgment and difficulties solving small problems. Mood changes, including irritation and mild anger spells, may also occur. Visio spatial problems such as judging distances are also possible, resulting in banging of the head or falling. Confusion about location often occurs, and difficulty remembering odd words. In addition headaches may become more frequent. There are various stages of dementia and in the early stages the difficulties encountered can be handled. Many people exist with dementia and live for up to twenty years or more, even after the dementia has become obvious. In the middle to latter stages Alzheimer's may well become apparent. However, with loving caregivers a reasonable quality of life can be maintained for quite a long time although the latter stages may prove difficult.

If you are over sixty five there is a 50% chance that you will have dementia. Many people, like myself, get progressively worse and are unaware that they actually have the condition, as many people regard poor memory and confusion as automatic in old age. In my own case I estimate that my dementia began when I was about sixty. It was not diagnosed for several years and because the advance of the disease was slow I was able to live a normal life and even write novels. Since changing my lifestyle the damage has almost stopped progressing, but the damage already done remains. This is limited to very poor memory for names and faces. Some difficulty remembering words and dealing with problems, such as the internet. More seriously my balance and judgment have deteriorated and I am more prone to tripping, stumbling and banging my head on things such as trees or awkward furniture. However, the advance has now almost stopped and my life is that of a normal healthy seventy two year old.

Although the statistics are scary, one should carry out a test on yourself, and if you think that you have dementia, consult your doctor as soon as possible. There may be a medical reason for your dementia that is treatable, such as a thyroid problem or vitamin deficiency.

Even if dementia is confirmed you must not fall into depression, but rather discuss it with family. Carry out research and take positive steps, it is possible to delay the progress of dementia and even arrest its advance. Think positively!

The simple test for dementia is to honestly answer the following questions. If you mostly answered 'Yes', consult your doctor for a thorough medical test and advice.

Do you suffer from short term memory loss?

Do you forget peoples' names?

Do you sometimes have difficulty with knowing where you are?

Do you have difficulties dealing with small problems such as banking or the internet?

Do you find that your balance is poor and that you trip or stumble?

Do you forget words?

The gift of knowledge will be a big help to you in dealing with dementia. Had I known at age sixty what I know now, I would have changed my life style and arrested the condition much earlier, resulting in less damage than has been done. So if you do have dementia don't rail against fate, know that you can change your lifestyle and slow down the advance of dementia or even stop it. Life with dementia is mainly a question of adjusting and you will probably be able to live an almost normal life, especially if you are able to avoid stress. You may even end up happier by dealing with your challenges.

'Wellbeing`, is a very important feature of dealing with dementia. This means not only exercises of mind and body and attention to diet and health, but also keeping a balanced state of mind. In my experience dementia patients suffer less from the medical condition, than other peoples' reaction! Those who have suddenly become poor will recollect how the people whom you expected to be sympathetic were often not so and the most unexpected people were kind and supportive. For some people poverty is deemed to be contagious and the same often applies to dementia and other illnesses, but one has to accept other peoples' failings and overcome the challenge and move from suffering to living. One interesting thing that I have learned is that nature often compensates and many dementia patients who have lost short term memory etc., actually become more intuitive. In fact in an article on 'The Alzheimer's Reading Room', there is a story about a man who was dying, entitled 'Man Living with Alzheimer's Predicts The Future.` It is the story of a man who told his daughter that she would get a certain job and other information and is quite fascinating.

After dementia has been medically diagnosed and Alzheimer's is the possible cause, it is time to start planning for the worst whilst still fighting for the best. The struggle involves dealing with depression and the loss of short term memory by practical steps. Apart from action to improve and maintain health of body, the mind and spirit must also be attended to.

Obviously a diary to write down things to do is the first step. The second, is the decision to tick the things when they are done, or you may forget that you have done them!

The early stages of memory loss and dementia are difficult to accept. It is very frustrating when you can't remember that word, or you forgot the shopping, or where you parked the car. Personally, when I can't remember a word the frustration almost hurts. However, I've found that if one goes through the alphabet looking for the word by its first letter, it often comes back. The other problems like shopping are not worth worrying about and keeping a diary helps tremendously.

So dementia really isn't the 'end of the world`; but you must understand that the condition is not only a challenge to you, but also to your loved ones. It takes time for even the best caregiver to understand that your annoying lapses in memory and odd moods and strange behaviour are not your fault, but rather that of your illness. You must be patient with them, as they will hopefully learn to be patient with you, and you will both come to know that the person inside is still you.

THIRD LETTER TO JULIAN

HOW BEST TO DEAL WITH DEMENTIA AND ALZHEIMER'S PATIENTS.

There is much advice available on this subject, but we found that some of the the most useful sources were 'Contented Dementia'; by Oliver James; and 'Learning To Speak Alzheimer's`; by Joanne Koenig Coste.

Although Oliver states in his 'Introduction` that his book is not intended for sufferers from dementia or Alzheimer's, but rather for the caregivers, I would recommend everyone to read it, regardless of which category you fall into.

James explains how Penny, a highly recognized caregiver, understood that 'Dementia sufferers have not lost their reason, just their short term memory. 'In the case discussed she explains that she knew that her patient had lost her recent information as to what she and Penny had been doing moments before. Penny recognized that the only difference between a dementia patient and other people, is that their memories lose the ability to store information efficiently. This does not happen overnight, but is a steady advance. In my own case, this has only partially happened before being almost arrested by the change of lifestyle and diet.

So to deal with the problem springing from the stress of trying to remember recent events, the caregiver must change the direction of the patient's memory, to happy memories or activities from their past.

The theory is based on the fact that dementia and Alzheimer's patients usually retain their long term memory, especially of things that they like to remember. To be effective, the caregiver needs to know something of the biography of the patient and a vivid imagination and the ability to discover and share the old memory. This has the effect of the patient feeling relaxed, contented and happy.

Penny's theory is that by making the effort to set the system in motion, the caregiver will not only help the patient by taking away the stress of trying to recall recent events, but also in due course lessen the caregivers task enormously. A wonderful investment of time for both.

Penny has three fundamental rules to enable the system to work.

1. Don't ask the patient questions.
2. Learn from them as the experts on their disability.
3. Always agree with them, never interrupt them.

Penny's system involves replacing normal 'common sense' that we use to communicate, with what she calls SPECALSENS. This means that we recognize that dementia sufferers lose most of their recent memories as the brain deteriorates, but retain memories from long ago, that are mostly complete and undamaged and we need to learn how to move the patient's thinking into the good memories.

To make these ideas work the caregiver needs to have the ability and courage to act out roles. Penny quotes an example of a male patient who suddenly dived under the table. She dropped something onto the floor to give herself an excuse to join him. She knew that he had been in

World War Two and assumed from the fact that he had his hands over his head that he was re-enacting a war time experience. She then joined him by role playing and said something like; "I think that it's all over now." She then continued with other assumed links and the patient quickly recovered and returned to the present, in a happy and pleased state.

The thing to be borne in mind with dementia patients is that for a lot of the time they are perfectly rational and coherent and often able to do most of the tasks of everyday living. It is the stress of trying to remember more recent events, or questions that they cannot deal with because of memory deficiency that can plunge them into despair and consequently strange and irrational behavior.

Caregivers need to remember that there is always a reason for irrational behavior by a patient and that to them the reaction to escape into the past is perfectly rational.

In 'Learning to Speak Alzheimer's', which was published much more recently, the advice and information goes further. It's subtitle could perhaps have been 'REALITY ORIENTATION VERSUS HABILATION.'

If dementia worsens and becomes Alzheimer's disease, or one of the other diseases of which dementia is the symptom, the patient's condition will change and worsen.

Short term memory will be badly affected, cognitive abilities will deteriorate and behavioral changes will take place.

In the past a policy of being blunt and 'honest' with patients was the accepted norm, this was known as 'Reality Orientation' and the consequences were endless confrontations between caregivers and patients and institutions seething with discontent or rows of 'vegetables' written off as lost. This incidentally was not only in the time of Charles Dickens, but continued up until a few years ago. Anyone suffering from 'senile dementia'or Alzheimer's disease was no longer human. Perhaps it is for this reason that so little progress has been made in finding a cure for Alzheimer's.

Because so little attention had been given to dealing with patients suffering from dementia and Alzheimer's, it was not consciously known or recognized that the causes of the difficulties experienced by patients were mainly that with very little short term memory, patients simply forget things. When they complain that they haven't been fed, it is usually because they have forgotten. If they repeatedly ask the same question, it is simply because they have forgotten that they asked the question before and what the answer was.

Because of memory, and difficulties in understanding they find questions stressful and often both beyond their comprehension and ability to respond.

In the past, the caregiver's response was often negative and confrontational. If for example an elderly patient said to a caregiver that she was going to visit her mother, who had been dead for many years, the caregiver's response would have been to be truthful and point out the reality with distressing consequences. This policy of 'Reality Orientation', was followed for a great many years. If the patient said that she 'wanted to go home', the caregiver would bluntly tell her that she couldn't, and a very distressed and agitated person was the consequence.

In her book 'Learning To Speak Alzheimer's', Joanne explains 'Habilation'. This is now recognized as being not only the most humane way of dealing with dementia and Alzheimer's patients, but also the most efficient. In simple terms the method is to divert the patient's improbable, or impossible objective by catching the patient's interest until such time as the original idea or intention is forgotten. So, to the lady wanting to visit her long dead mother one might say; "Tell me about that." Or, "Tell me about your mother." If possible they would look at photographs and hopefully bring back happy memories, because so much long term memory is often retained.

In response to someone 'Wanting To Go Home', one might say; "Let's go and chose something to wear." Or' "You could wear your green shirt". Or red dress etc. It should be borne in mind that 'home' to an Alzheimer's patient can mean several things and not necessarily the last home that they lived in. It may mean that they long for the security they experienced as a child in a specific home. Or it could mean somewhere else that they have lived in, or it could just mean that they are feeling insecure. In all cases, diversion to happier and more contented thoughts or memories is the best procedure.

To some, the idea of diverting patients objectives by this method may sound dishonest, but morally one's duty is to act in the patient's best interest and to keep him or her happy is the kindest and also most efficient route to follow. Although dealing with patients in this way calls for more effort and the ability to think quickly and imaginatively, in the long run it will also alleviate the caregiver's burden, because the method will flow automatically with practice.

Apart from not confronting patients with the 'truth', appropriate body language must also be employed and the voice used in a gentle manner. Alzheimer's patients tend to focus on the speaker's eyes and 'read' meaning through eye contact and so caregivers need to give special attention to this fact.

Body language in general is very important to patients, and so it is not sufficient to just deflect questions, the skill of 'Habilation' must be thought about and learned. The voice must be warm and friendly, the caregiver must face the patient and speak slowly and bear in mind that patients lose much of their memory of vocabulary, so sentences should be short and simple.

FOURTH LETTER TO JULIAN

WHAT IS ALZHEIMERS?

Dear Julian ,Having worked with me researching Alzheimer's, you are aware of all the points that follow, but for others this may be a first encounter and clarify the situation. Much more detailed information can be found on the internet.

Research indicates that Alzheimer's disease is associated with plaques and tangles in the brain. The effect of the disease is to slowly destroy the brain cells, resulting in loss of memory, cognitive difficulties in solving problems and ultimately death because the brain will eventually cease to send the messages to the body in respect of breathing and death will result. Death may occur before this, because of chronic illness.

However, research shows that Alzheimer's is not inevitable because of old age. Much depends on heredity as well as health and life style. Researchers have discovered a gene regulator active during fetal brain development, called REST. This is either lost over the years or remains dormant and if dormant it appears to remove the risk of Alzheimer's disease in later life.

Alzheimer's patients have been known to live for twenty years and in the early stages which are heralded by the symptom which is dementia, a fairly normal life can be led. In my own case I am in the second stage of dementia and yet I am writing this book. Although the advance of my dementia has been almost stopped, the previous damage remains. This results in some short term memory loss and a little loss of long term memory. Remembering peoples' names, or sometimes if they are only acquaintances even their faces, is a big problem, as is remembering travel routes or directions. Also, I sometimes struggle for words, but they usually come back after a concentrated mental effort. In addition my orientation is impaired and I sometimes trip or bang by head. The last point is actually the most serious at the moment because it requires one to be careful because of the danger of injury. However, I walk and swim, read, write and enjoy my life very much.

However, if my dementia were to advance and Alzheimer's to take over in the years to come, then the following may happen. Because the brain cells are slowly being destroyed the memory will gradually deteriorate considerably and may reach the point where the identity of even the caregiver may be intermittent. This is of course a terrible problem for relatives and loved ones and not surprisingly many discontinue visiting once the patient is in a Care Home. However, we now know that the person is still inside, it is not just a vegetable slumped there and with knowledge and love they can be reached, in effect they are just asleep.

Alzheimer patients need a caregiver who is a friend who cares and can learn incredible patience. Apart from the steady advance of the illness boredom is an enemy. Social intercourse should be continued and dignity and preserved until the very end. For the 'aware' patient this is very important, as many elderly people become incontinent. Even those who are not aware deserve dignity.

The caregiver must learn to read body movements in order to understand the needs and wants of the patient, because speech deteriorates and may even disappear.

Caregivers must not despair sometimes of being a caregiver, although such feelings are perfectly natural and being a caregiver will seem almost unbearable at times. The early stages of Alzheimer's are difficult, but the latter can be heartbreaking and it is for this reason that it is worth investing time in understanding the disease and the positive steps that can be taken to slow the advance.

FIFTH LETTER TO JULIAN

WELCOME TO ALZHEIMER'S WORLD

Dear Julian, it seems so strange to write those words. After all, what could possibly be welcoming about the world of Alzheimer's disease. However, if one advances from the dementia stage to Alzheimer's one has moved on into a new and challenging world. The only way that the caregiver can positively help their loved one is to understand and share that world.

To look after a loved one who is suffering from dementia or Alzheimer's will call for an enormous investment of time. In the early stages it will be very time consuming, but probably not too difficult, as the memory loss will possibly be small and further deterioration only gradual and by being watchful, can be dealt with.

The reduction in cognitive abilities is a slightly bigger problem that calls for patience in sorting things out, that the patient now has difficulties with. In my own case, as you know, I now need help with computer difficulties, but so do lots of older people, so it isn't really such a drama. This is where grandchildren can be useful.

Although dementia and Alzheimer's can be slowed down, or even stopped with the steps already outlined, sadly there is as yet no going back. The portion of the brain already damaged will remain so and the difficulties with short term memory loss already experienced, will remain at that level. However, to stop further deterioration will be a tremendous achievement. Even slowing deterioration down will extend the quality of life.

The term 'Alzheimer's World' was the idea of Bob Del Marco of 'The Alzheimer's Reading Rooms.' This is an excellent source of information and was created by Bob because he looked after his mother Dotty.

Bob struggled as all caregivers of an Alzheimer patient do with persistent questions and aggressive and rude and hostile behavior from his mother. Eventually he realized that Dotty couldn't change her behavior, but he could change his understanding and approach. He knew that to do this he would need to understand the world in which the Alzheimer victim inhabits and how to step inside and almost be able to speak a new language.

Understanding the cause of patient's difficult behavior was the first step and this really almost totally came down to memory loss and the stress of trying to understand questions and what was happening.

Bob realized that an Alzheimer's patient saw the 'outside' world through different eyes. He realized that it was frightening and threatening to not always understand what was happening.

Bob's approach was to first smile and then to speak slowly and calmly to Dotty and to use as few words as possible. Alzheimer's patients are often only able to understand one word in four. When Dotty left the fridge door open, he realized that she had just forgotten to close it. When she asked repeated questions, she had just forgotten the answers. When she claimed that she hadn't been fed, he realized that she had just forgotten .Bob learned patience and because of his love and new understanding the relationship changed from one of conflict into a happy one.

Another source of information for me was Joe Huey of alzheimerhope.com who set out a useful list of ten rules for dealing with a dementia or Alzheimer patient.

TEN RULES FOR DEALING WITH DEMENTIA AND ALZHEIMER'S PATIENTS

1. Never argue   always agree
2. Never reason   instead divert

3. Never shame	instead distract
4. Never lecture	instead re-assess
5. Never say; 'remember'	instead reminisce
6. Never say; 'I told you'	instead repeat
7. Never say; 'You can't'	instead find out what
8. Never demand or command	instead ask, or be a model
9. Never condescend	instead encourage or praise
10. Never force	instead reinforce gently

As a caregiver you have a rocky road ahead, dementia and Alzheimer's call for a lot of knowledge, patience and understanding, but there will be lots of joy ahead as well, and no matter how hard there is always hope. Patience is also needed, but if one can master the way to understand patients and divert where necessary, there will be a reward in the form of an easier relationship between the caregiver and the patient in the future. Welcome to Alzheimer's World!

SIXTH LETTER TO JULIAN

THE PROOF OF LOVE

Love does make a difference to a person suffering from dementia or Alzheimer's. The early stages of dementia are not too difficult to understand. They call for patience and kindness. At least the patient can still communicate and conversations and memory sharing can take place.

In our particular case we have discussed and investigated what may happen and the possibilities to come. We have both been blessed with a very positive attitude.

The latter stages of Alzheimer's are much more difficult, not only because the patient is much more confused and even sometimes abusive, but also because the sufferer seems to have gone and just a living shell remains. However, we now know that this is often not the case and the patient inside can often be reached by music, touching and patient love.

In a way the latter stages are perhaps the most important for caregivers to understand. Certainly for the patient, they must be the most painful, and love must reach them and they not be emotionally abandoned.

Love is the key and with love the advance of both dementia and Alzheimer's can be delayed. With enough love and patience they can be dramatically delayed.

It is sadly recorded that in experiments carried out by the Nazis on babies, they fed the children well and cared for them in every medical and physical way, but totally deprived them of any love or affection. They were completely ignored in a loving way and deprived emotionally. They all died.

Love given really works, but love denied can break the spirit.

SEVENTH LETTER TO JULIAN

HUMOUR IS MEDICATION

Thank you for all the humour and laughter that you have brought into my life .A smile is the first step to laughter. Laughter has been proved to be a positive medicine. Your patient should, dependent on the stage of the illness be treated to jokes and humour. A happy emotional state will benefit the patient enormously and help to slow down the onset of Alzheimer's, rather like positive thinking improves health. So keep smiling!

Don't take it personally if the patient becomes a 'handful`, or in my case an even bigger 'handful`! Try and move on emotionally and remember that the person inside is still the same, they just act differently because of the disease.

EIGHTH LETTER TO JULIAN

DEMENTIA, ALZHEIMERS AND COMMUNICATION

When dealing with a person suffering from Dementia or Alzheimer's, communication is essential and it sometimes takes a special skill to communicate with a person suffering from either, but this is especially true of Alzheimer's.

The effect of the disease is predominantly to damage the brain and thus the memory and cognitive abilities. This means that the patient is existing in an inner world without the benefit of these faculties apart from on a reduced basis. It is hardly surprising therefore that the person feels frustration with their reduced abilities to remember recent events, problem solve and even to communicate. This is often expressed in anger, or even aggression. From my own experience I can say that it almost hurts when you strain to remember something that just eludes one.

The caregiver has to understand that memory loss means that you forget what you have recently been told and you may even have forgotten that you have recently eaten. Imagine how frustrating it must be to forget so many things, even sometimes who your loved ones are. You are the same person inside, you just forget things and can't always solve simple problems .You have to understand that this leaves the person in great difficulty and the only way to fully understand and to communicate is for you to step into 'Alzheimer's World.' This means learning to understand how to communicate in that special way. Learning how to smile and look the person in the eyes and speak gently. Learning how to control your own natural feelings of annoyance and irritation, and how to hide them. Learning how to communicate, in the world of dementia and Alzheimer's.

If like myself you are a dementia sufferer already, understanding your own challenges will be easier if you understand the problems of others more advanced along the 'rocky road' than yourself. Understanding is everything and you can arrest or slow down the pace of your own dementia by understanding the challenges of others.

With the gift of knowledge you can practice the exercise of body, mind and spirit. Fight depression and be positive. Visualize yourself relaxed, happy and still with your current faculties in ten or twenty years.

NINTH LETTER TO JULIAN

FOLLOWING

As Alzheimer's patients increasingly become dependent on their caregiver, there is often a tendency to follow the carergiver around. Whilst this is a little tiresome, it isn't usually an enormous problem. However, everyone needs privacy sometimes, even if it's just to go to the loo!

The cause of following, is a feeling of dependency on the caregiver and insecurity when they are not there. The solution to this difficulty is for the caregiver to give the patient an explanation each time that she leaves the room. The explanations need to be simple and understandable to the patient. "I'm just going to put the kettle" or "hang out the washing."

The objective is to get the patient used to the fact that when the caregiver leaves the room it isn't forever and that there is no threat to the relationship.

TENTH LETTER TO JULIAN

DEMENTIA AND CHRISTMAS

The holidays are a time when friends and family often spend time together. For the family living with dementia or Alzheimer disease the holidays can seem very challenging.

With early or middle stage dementia sufferers the challenges can be met and the holidays enjoyed. It is a good idea to explain to visitors in advance of their arrival, either by telephone or perhaps by letter or e mail that the loved one has dementia. Explain the manifestations of the dementia, such as the memory loss, which may include them, their names and their faces. Explain that the person may repeat questions and explain the reason, which is memory loss etc.

Ask that they remain very calm and very patient and try to bear in mind that the person is the same inside, it is just the illness that may make them behave differently.

Family reunions are often emotional and fraught. But, if explained properly, very often the presence of a dementia sufferer can in fact even bring the family closer together, so don't be stressed about the prospect, relax and think positively.

ELEVENTH LETTER TO JULIAN

INFECTION, FALLING AND OTHER DANGERS

Apart from infections caused by bed sores, which need to be avoided by watchful care, bladder infections are also a big problem with patients.

Not only can infection be a great risk to Alzheimer and Dementia patients, but can in addition be a source of bad behavior. Thus caregivers must be watchful that difficult behavior is not a sign of a health problem.

However, falling is a big problem to sufferers of both dementia and Alzheimer Disease and leads to many injuries and deaths. Falling or tripping or the banging of the head can be caused by the disorientation and poor balance caused by Alzheimer's brain damage.

Another danger is that patients sometimes put things into their mouths, so constant vigilance is needed to safeguard the person.

TWELTH LETTER TO JULIAN

WANDERING AND HOW TO REDUCE THE RISKS

A large number of people in late stage Dementia and also many with Alzheimer Disease 'escape' their caregivers and wander off. Most are quickly found, but those that are not found quickly are at enormous risk and many, are never found. The statistics, for those who wander in the United States make sad reading.

Of those found within two to twelve hours only 93% survive. After 24 hours, only one third are found alive and after 72 hours only one in five are found alive.

These terrible statistics illustrate just how vulnerable dementia and Alzheimer's patients are. They are of course more prone to accidents and to become victims of crime, when in 'Alzheimer's World` as they often don't respond when spoken to.

As always, there is some good news and that is that most Alzheimer patients are found within a mile of home.

A good idea to reduce the risk of danger is to persuade the person to wear one of those silver or chromium identity bracelets with name, address and caregiver's telephone number. In addition, there are some very good tracking devices available that have alert facilities that can be triggered if the patient leaves the garden or grounds.

In the early stages of dementia wandering off will not be such a problem, but in the later stages, serious thought will have to be given to this challenge.

THIRTEENTH LETTER TO JULIAN

DEMENTIA AND ALZHEIMERS---BLAME GRANDPA

At the time of writing in 2014 the number of Alzheimer victims in the United Kingdom is approaching one million and in the United States over five million and the reasons for Alzheimer's disease are increasingly being sought. One reason however, is statistics. People are living longer therefore there are more of them, including more Alzheimer victims. The reasons for improved longevity are predominantly better medical care.

It has been fashionable to blame the passive watching of television as one reason for dementia. The truth is not that simple. There is for example a big difference between watching a nature program and a film with gratuitous violence and also the amount of time spent watching television. Too much TV is almost certainly a negative, no matter how good the content. In addition Alzheimer patients in the later stages are sometimes very influenced by television and can become delusional and believe that they are the characters in a film or 'soapy' and can even be violent.

There is no doubt that an active lifestyle helps to reduce the probability of dementia. The reason is fairly straight forward, in that good health is as beneficial to the brain as it is to the heart. However, in the case of dementia physical exercise through walking, sport or gym is not enough. The brain must also be used;-statistics show that reading, studying, dealing with mental challenges and social involvement, reduce the chances of Alzheimer's. In fact, even playing computer games are believed to be beneficial to memory, although there are suggestions that some of the more anti social games where violence and theft are part have a negative effect on both young and old.

However, research also shows that heredity also plays a part in mental health, so check out Grandpa and Grandma as well, if you have dementia it may not be entirely your fault!

Although there is nothing that you can do about your heredity, it is helpful to know if there is a history of dementia, as it can be a warning and encourage a good life style. At the time of writing there is no test to show if one has Alzheimer's, or even a pre disposition to the disease, but there are indications that this will change in the very near future.

FOURTEENTH LETTER TO JULIAN

BLAME THE DISEASE AND NOT THE PERSON

IF dementia gets worse and Alzheimer's is revealed, your loved one may become more difficult. This is of course because of the steady damage to the brain. The time scale varies enormously. Some books claim that with Alzheimer's one will live for another three to nine years after diagnosis. However, my research shows that if you include the dementia period, patients can live for thirty years or more. In fact in my own case I now realize that I have had dementia for about ten years and yet I have been able to live a normal life and the symptoms have now almost stopped advancing. However, it is often the case that the dementia patient becomes more difficult as the illness progresses. Patients change in different ways and caregivers must focus on what is left and not what is lost. The approach to your loved one must be to smile and greet and reach through the veil into 'Alzheimer's World`, the mental 'space' in which Alzheimer patients inhabit.

It is common for Alzheimer's patients to start to lose vocabulary and by the middle stage they may have lost words and may only understand every fourth word. Thus one must speak in a simple way; keep sentences very short and speak slowly and allow a gap between sentences for the patient to absorb and understand.

Often patients will talk about a third party; " Bobby wants a drink of water." They mean themselves and the caregiver must understand this and almost speak as if to a baby. This is difficult for the caregiver to deal with, as of course pity for the loved one or patient, will naturally be felt. However, it was perhaps harder for the patient at the earlier stages because of the awareness of what is happening to one. Before my dementia almost stopped advancing it was often dispiriting to realize that memories were fading and would probably never return.

At the earlier stages of dementia the loved one is rational for most of the time and normal discourse can take place, however in the more advanced stages rational discussion will be very difficult. At these later stages the art of diversion becomes essential. Questions from the patient are often repeated, because they have forgotten the earlier answer. Sometimes they will claim that they are hungry or aren't being fed. This is not to be difficult, it will be because they don't remember. It has been suggested that one way to deal with this particular problem is to divide the meal into two or more portions, to make it easier for caregiver.

Conflict must be avoided at all times and the caregiver will avoid complicated explanations and use the art of diversion and perhaps encourage the patient to do something different, such as a walk or to play a game. It is important to also remember that with the progressive brain damage the patient loses empathy and doesn't always mean what he says. Rude and cutting things must be ignored and diversion practiced. The caregiver must be aware in advance of the changes that may come and how they will deal with the challenges.

For caregivers with the loved one at home, it is essential that as many family members as possible are involved in the caring. They must all be aware of the fact that the real person is still inside. They must be encouraged to share some of the workload to give the principal caregiver breaks. It must be a joint and shared operation.

There will be memory difficulties at all stages. To help your loved one remember faces or names, try to jog their memory by talking about the person and perhaps tell a story about the past in which the person features.

It is now known that Alzheimer patients can be reached even in the last stages of Alzheimer disease, so they are never beyond hope, help or love.

Perhaps the hardest thing for caregivers is not to take the things that advanced Alzheimer patients say to heart. It will require planning to be ready for these challenges when they come. However, it could be many years from when dementia is first diagnosed. Above all, caregivers must try not to get angry with the patient because of rude or aggressive behavior. It is their disease that has damaged their brain that is speaking.

As time goes on, communication and understanding will become more difficult. Caregivers should be aware that sometimes body movement replaces speech. So one should take an interest in what the patient is doing. Everything means something. If the loved one bangs on the table, perhaps he wants attention. If you don't understand the word that the patient is using, ask an obscure sentence, such as; "Let's have a cup of tea;'". "Let's go for a walk" ; etc. Caregivers must be prepared to be patient. Practice taking deep breaths before answering questions.

Sometimes, reactions to colours, sounds, smells tastes and even changes in temperature, can put the loved one back into the past. Sometimes they will be happy memories and sometimes sad. Try and empathize with the patient and draw them out and if necessary divert them to happy memories.

Although some memories may be distressing, they may actually help the patient, because they are remembering which can be good. Also, some will remember their achievements in life, in their work or business or raising a family. Everyone wants to feel that they are respected, admired and of course still loved and wanted. So talking and listening and sharing music, can help a person to deal with the effects of Alzheimer's. Music especially, can be very soothing.

Sometimes memory will come back to a surprising degree as memory loss is a grey area. It feels a bit like living in a mist that lifts and descends. Caregivers must show patience and an interest if the person becomes even temporarily lucid.

Caregivers must also be on the look out for the causes of distress. Apart from the bewilderment of memory loss, patients may be experiencing actual physical difficulties, such as pain, constipation or illness. Sometimes a worsening in speech and memory can mean delirium, which can be caused by an infection. Caregivers need to be constantly watchful and of course a doctor called for advice, if worries about the patient persist.

Looking after a person suffering from dementia or Alzheimer disease is a very focused task. Even in the early stages of dementia when the loved one is still compos mentis, a watchful eye will have to be kept in case the person trips or falls and also forgetfulness, such as leaving doors open can be sometimes very disruptive. Later on, the task will become harder and in addition to all the care required, a caregiver will need to see that the loved one or patient is stimulated. For as long as it is possible, walking for example is an excellent way to keep the senses alive. If possible it is so much better if accompanied, and indeed in many cases this will of course be essential. Trips out are an adventure for anyone who doesn't get out very often and visits to friends and relatives are very good therapy, or even just a drive in the country. For some, a visit to McDonalds would be a great treat.

However, even sitting in the garden if weather permits will be rewarding to many. Just listening to the birds and watching the clouds move across the sky . This may well also give the caregiver a bit of a break if circumstances permit. Many people also find that a pet such as a dog can be very beneficial to someone who is unwell and if possible this should be encouraged.

In the early stages of dementia we don't need a great deal of attention, but if Alzheimer's is reached then this will change. It will be important to ensure that the loved one or patient continues to be active both bodily and mentally. Television should not be watched excessively and talking, singing, playing games, music and if possible regular humor should all be enjoyed. Make jokes whenever possible. Some care homes are supported by volunteers who call in on a weekly basis and in many cases involve the patients in zany humor. It is strongly believed by the staff in those homes involved, that this helps tremendously in slowing down the advance of Alzheimer disease.

FIFTEENTH LETTER TO JULIAN

DEMENTIA AND ALZHEIMERS – TAKING MEDICATIONS

Sometimes patients can be difficult, or even refuse to take medication. It is always important to remember not to confuse patients by explaining too much. This can lead to confusion and confrontations and a refusal to do what you want.

First, look them in the eye and as always smile and offer the medication, one pill at a time. If you give them a glass of water, use a small glass that is easier to hold. After they have taken the glass, offer the pill on the palm of your hand. Try and say nothing and usually they will react from habit and take the pill. The same principal applies with liquid medication. If they refuse to take their medication, stop and try again a little later.

Afterwards, if it is morning give them a cup of tea or coffee and talk to them gently so that they remember that with 'pill taking' there will follow a sort of reward. If it is evening you might offer cocoa.

If swallowing pills is a problem, check with the doctor or pharmacist if the medication can be taken any other way, for example crushed and mixed with yogurt or food.

It is also a good idea to keep a list of medications and discuss with the doctor or pharmacist if there are any side effects and also confirm that the various medications are compatible. In addition, it is important to know the time of day when each medication should be taken and if before or after meals. Sometimes medicines can have side effects such as constipation, so this has to be considered and the appropriate dietary steps taken.

Caregivers are only human, so it is important to either keep a calendar and tick off when medications have been given or use a pill box organizer.

SIXTEENTH LETTER TO JULIAN

GASLIGHTING AND DEMENTIA

It is possible for most people to live an almost normal life in the early to middle stages of dementia. The time scale depends of course at what speed the dementia is advancing. If the caregiver ensures that the loved one keeps healthy and active the advance may be slow. However, in the latter stages of dementia the underlying Alzheimer's can be utterly destructive. To those of a certain age close to my own, the word 'Gaslight' will ring a bell and they may even remember as I do, my parents mentioning this film. It was released in 1934 and starred Ingrid Bergman.

The story is based in the days when house lighting was by gas. In the film a husband tries to drive his wife insane by playing tricks with the gas lighting and carries out strange manifestations, which he pretends only she can see. The relevance of this today is that it is not uncommon for Alzheimer's patients to believe that their caregivers are lying to them, robbing them and other dastardly deeds and this phenomenon is known as 'gas lighting`.

The way to deal with this problem is not to argue with the patient, but rather to empathize and divert. For example, if accused of stealing something the caregiver might say ;"Oh I'm so sorry about this, let me help you find it."

Always remember that you cannot debate rationally with an Alzheimer's patient. Do not be afraid that you are encouraging the person's irrational belief, just be sympathetic and if something is misplaced, help them to find it.

The difficult behavior of Alzheimer's patients is caused by emotional or physical issues. Loss of control of their lives is of course a big reason and the reaction of anger and paranoia is not so surprising when you consider the 'drowning feeling` that loss of memory and cognitive abilities creates. In addition, there may be medical reasons and a watchful eye must be kept for illness, discomfort, or problems with medications.

To actually deal with the gas lighting problem is immensely difficult and of course the 'bad behavior ', and often nastiness do not endear the patient to the caregiver or relatives. However, understanding is everything. One must focus on what is happening to the loved one and ignore the bad manifestations. It is very, very hard and of course being a caregiver is not easy and calls for great depths of understanding and love, but imagine the loneliness of the patient, trapped in a sort of fog.

However, it should never be forgotten that whilst most complaints by Alzheimer's patients are groundless, there might just be occasionally a genuine complaint, so a watchful eye must always be maintained.

THE SEVENTEENTH LETTER TO JULIAN

SUNDOWNING

Even when dementia has not yet manifested into Alzheimer's, ' sundowning` may happen. This, as the name implies is a phenomenon of the late afternoon or early evening, when the sun goes down. The manifestations are aggression, agitation, delusions, paranoia ,increased disorientation and wandering.

Where sundowning is apparent, increased exercise, no caffeine after lunch and the presence of a nightlight as dusk descends can help. Care should focus on optimizing an individual's health and quality of life and if the loved one is still at home other family members should reduce the pressure on the principal caregiver. Diverting the patient in the late afternoon with other activities will also help.

Presumably the movement of the sun effects us all, but like the full moon phenomenon it only manifests in certain individuals, but is common with those people with our illness.

THE EIGHTEENTH LETTER TO JULIAN

DEMENTIA --- THE MIDDLE STAGES

The middle stages of dementia are typically the longest and can last for many years. As a dementia sufferer myself and still in the early stages and in remission, I hope that if my dementia does advance again it will not go beyond the middle stages. If it does so, I hope that there will not be sufficient deterioration that I will need to go into a care home. However, in most cases of Alzheimer's at the last stages, it is probably much kinder for the patient to be in an environment where a high level of care is available.

As Alzheimer's disease manifests itself in the middle dementia stages, the challenge of the earlier stages will become bigger. The earlier memory loss will have grown worse, although not necessarily so bad that the caregivers are forgotten, although intermittently this may happen.

There may be greater difficulties with words and speech, expression, and words may be jumbled. There may also now be some difficulties in dressing, frustration and anger and slight anti social behavior, such as a reluctance to bathe.

A caregiver at this stage of dementia will need even greater patience than before and even greater knowledge of dementia and what to expect, but with love, skill and perhaps a little luck the challenge will not be any more overwhelming. The caregiver, will through experience have acquired the knowledge and developed the skill needed to deal with the loved one with whom they are entrusted.

The first thing to remember is always have a smiling face. Sometimes this will be difficult, but it really is worthwhile. Sometimes, a dementia sufferer will be in a fog and perhaps not understand where they are, or who they are. A smiling face and a gentle voice will re-assure. Remember the ten rules for dealing with dementia and Alzheimer's patients. Learn to divert and never to argue. Never force; beguile and persuade, or defer until a better opportunity presents itself.

The middle dementia years are usually manageable with love, patience and a lot of energy! The loved one can probably still be part of the family and once family members are used to the situation, everyone can participate in the caring . Responsibilities can and indeed must be shared and the principal caregiver allowed and encouraged to take breaks from the hard task of looking after a dementia patient.

NINETEENTH LETTER TO JULIAN

DEMENTIA AND SLEEPING

Many people experience difficulties with sleeping, and with age this usually gets worse and evidence suggests that dementia and Alzheimer patients experience this problem even more than others. Being one of the insomniacs myself I have much sympathy for others. Although I am not sure if sleeping pills are harmful or not, I have to admit that rather than toss and turn for many hours and then feel 'hung over' the next day, I take a pill myself.

Interestingly, many long lived people in good health state that they sleep easily for between seven and eight hours and have always done so. So sleep is important. Good health in all aspects seems to be very relevant to fighting dementia and Alzheimer's and in addition the ability to ' switch off' and learn to deal with stress. Also, having an enjoyable occupation and a good partner seem to contribute to longevity and reduce the chances of dementia and Alzheimer's. However, if the probability of these two demons is in our genes then our task in dealing with them is much more difficult.

In my own case my mother I now realize had dementia and very probably Alzheimer's but my father didn't and died at a good age of other causes. So my chances of the diseases coming partially from heredity are fifty fifty. However, my past life style would have encouraged the probability and I suspect contributed to insomnia. Now that I live a more balanced lifestyle with no alcohol or smoking and a very healthy diet my sleeping has become better.

Difficulty in sleeping is very common with the elderly and also there is a reduction in dreaming, although there doesn't appear to be a link between this and the quality of sleep.

The problem for caregivers is that those patients who have dementia and Alzheimer's and difficulty in sleeping may call out and disturb caregivers. They may also wander around and put themselves at risk.

TWENTIETH LETTER TO JULIAN

DEMENTIA AND PAIN

There is no pain specific to dementia, but up to 50% of elderly patients, experience pain. However, the pain experienced by elderly people of age sixty or over is unrelated to either dementia or Alzheimer's. Pain is commonly caused by rheumatoid arthritis, cancer symptoms, colon problems etc.

Caregivers must be watchful for pain and seek appropriate medical advice and treatment. This is particularly important when the patient can no longer fully communicate, especially those suffering from Alzheimer's disease.

TWENTY FIRST LETTER TO JULIAN

DEMENTIA AND DRIVING

Those still in the early stages of dementia can usually continue to drive. Legal requirements vary in different countries, but both the caregiver and the patient should be watchful. Once disorientation becomes a feature of the dementia driving should cease, both in the interest of the patient, the passengers and other road users. In my particular case I am still driving, but I know Julian that you have some doubts about this; but then 'no man is a driving hero to his wife'!

TWENTY SECOND LETTER TO JULIAN

DEMENTIA AND DANGER

A normal home has many dangers to a dementia or Alzheimer's patient and precautions must be taken. Obstacles to trip over, slippery floors or loose rugs should be dealt with. Kitchen utensils, things cooking or boiling etc. can also be a problem. Water temperatures of showers or baths should obviously not be too high and a watch kept on the patient to ensure that they are aware before they step into the bath or under the shower. Locks should be removed from locks on toilet or bathroom doors and open fires guarded.

However, subject to a watchful eye, patients should be encouraged wherever possible to continue with non dangerous activities and visits out encouraged, subject to careful accompaniment.

TWENTY THIRD LETTER TO JULIAN

DIFFICULTY SWALLOWING

Many late stage dementia and Alzheimer's patients have difficulty swallowing. This is mainly because they have forgotten how to swallow, or sometimes even how to chew.

The symptoms, can be coughing whilst eating, because sometimes the food goes down the wrong way and gets caught in the airways. It is essential that the caregiver is watchful for this, not only because of the risk of choking, but also because food gets caught in the throat.

According to Bob Del Marco of 'The Alzheimer's Reading Rooms', if the food gets caught and trapped, this can lead to Pulmonary Choking. This means the entry of food into the tract and lungs and can be fatal as it can lead to pneumonia.

Caregivers need to be very watchful for the risk of choking. Sometimes patients will put too much food into their mouth and the results can be fatal.

TWENTY FOURTH LETTER TO JULIAN

MEMORY COMES AND GOES

Julian, you will remember the time that we attended your aunt's ninetieth birthday party. It was a huge party and relatives had come from all over South Africa, but when we arrived the poor lady was not very well and in bed. She appeared to have totally lost her memory and you were very worried about her as she certainly appeared to be suffering from late stage Alzheimer's.

Frankly, things look bad, but the next day a relative contacted you to say that "Auntie is now right as rain." She was up and about and disappointed that she had missed her party. She was carrying out her daily chores and hopefully, like other of your relatives she has a good few years to look forward to.

This was very thought provoking to me, as I had feared the worst and not imagined that the lady's memory would return. I should have known better, because my own memory loss is not constant. Most days are fine, but sometimes I forget names, faces and words and on others my memory is more productive.

Dementia in the early stages does not stop victims from living an almost normal life. Sometimes struggling for words is frustrating, but the words usually come back when you focus, although the effort required can I find be rather exhausting. Although with dementia and Alzheimer's some long term memories will be lost, mostly it is an intermittent problem and it is short term memory retention that is the serious challenge.

It is also worth mentioning that patients should be encouraged to look after themselves as much as possible, as your aunt has done. The more occupied that patients are, the better their memory challenges can be overcome.

TWENTY FIFTH LETTER TO JULIAN

DEMENTIA AND DENIAL

This letter is about something that we have discussed many times. Because memory loss is such a significant feature of dementia Alzheimer's; patients find it difficult when caregivers or others, tell them about the things that they have, or haven't done and we are tempted to disbelieve you. This is certainly true of myself as it is very hard to accept the 'blanks' in our memories. The professionals say that patients should not be stressed about these things and they are usually best left unsaid.

My dementia, I now realize has been with me for about ten years. It began with forgetting names and faces and as it grew slowly worse over the years, from time to time I would visit the doctor and emerge reassured that at least it wasn't Alzheimer's.

When finally my condition was diagnosed as dementia I was prompted to investigate my condition. The revelation that dementia is the symptom of something worse, and probably Alzheimer's was quite a shock that propelled me to look for ways to stop the advance of the disease.

After changing my lifestyle to a Mediterranean diet, stopping the whisky, brandy and wine and also the cigars, my health improved dramatically and is now better than for many years. Although I knew from my research that one couldn't 'turn back the clock' on memory loss, I had at least had slowed down my memory loss and almost stopped the advance.

It was the revelation that in fact I was still forgetting recent events that brought home the fact that although I had certainly slowed down the progress of the disease, I had not stopped it totally.

This was a terrible shock to me, but apparently denial is very usual at the early stage of the disease, both by the victim and the caregiver. However, in due course I came to terms with my situation. Reflecting on my life, my blessings were so apparent that I could only count my blessings in so many ways.

Perhaps the recognition of denial is a step that we must all go through and accept that it is not what we have lost that now matters, but we have left.

TWENTY SIXTH LETTER TO JULIAN

EATING PROBLEMS? TRY RED PLATES

`Sometimes dementia or Alzheimer's patients don't want to eat. Often it is simple things that put the patients off their food. Perhaps the food is too hot, or too cold, or the patient has chewing difficulties. Dentures should be checked in case chewing is painful and also glasses should be worn as food is visual as well as about taste.

Depression and dehydration are also sometimes causes of lack of appetite. Perhaps the patient needs more exercise. Other causes might be constipation, or a lack of variety in the food. Research has also shown that regular small meals are better than a few big ones.

Finally, it is apparently a fact that red plates encourage the appetite! In our house lack of appetite was never a problem, but this might be a useful fact to know.

TWENTY SEVENTH LETTER TO JULIAN

DEMENTIA PATIENTS HOW TO REMEMBER BETTER

Before reaching the latter stages of dementia it is possible to fight to retain short term memory for as long as possible and hopefully these memories may be retained; even though later on this may not be the case. It is easier to remember what we are interested in, or what has affected us deeply. Thus we can remember songs and bits of poetry without much effort. I have

50

found that if I look for something interesting about what I want to remember, then I can usually remember, but of course it does require effort. For example, to remember people's faces look for special features, such as beautiful eyes, a big nose, a scar, a wart etc. To remember peoples' names try and think of something amusing to link the name to. Take 'John` for example. There used to be a TV series about an American Hillbilly family called 'The Waltons`. At the end of each program the characters would be in bed ready for sleep. They would call out 'Good night' to one another. The principal character was John whose uncle also shared the same name and so the last dialogue of the show was "Good night uncle John"; and the shouted reply was ; "Good night John boy." Association is all that is called for. All names can be linked to something, so if John's name was Smith one could visualize a shoe smith with a forge and big hammer hitting read hot horse shoes into shape. If the surname was 'Walton`, you might remember 'a walled town' and so on.

It is also definitely easier to remember rhyming things. For example in Cockney slang 'stairs' are 'apples and pears'.; a suit is a 'whistle and flute.'

Another memory method which is also linked to humour is to remember names by silly opposites. So Mr. Goode would be Mr. Bad. Someone called Jerry could be remembered by thinking of a 'Jerry can', which is a petrol container, or Jerry Lee Lewis, who only those of a certain age will remember.

Personally, I remember images more easily than words or numbers. For example, if I am trying to remember an address I visualize the house and the name usually comes back. I find that the sillier the association, the easier the word is to remember. So if I am shopping I would remember the following. 'Bread-Dead'. 'Butter-Nutter'. 'Dog food-Hog food'.etc.

The possibilities are endless and quite good fun as well!

TWENTY EIGHTH LETTER TO JULIAN

LET THE DEMENTIA PATIENT CONTINUE NORMALLY IF POSSIBLE

In the early stages of dementia, many patients can still carry out most every day tasks, such as driving, shopping etc. Once the reality of the doctor's diagnosis has sunk in, it is often the instinct of the caregiver to do as much as possible for the loved one.

However, for as long as patients can carry out routine tasks they should be encouraged to do so, as this will help them retain their cognitive abilities. As time goes on, many tasks will become joint efforts, such as banking and the family finances, but the input of the patient should be treasured for as long as possible.

It is also at this stage that caregivers sometimes clutch at straws and hope that the dementia is not real and perhaps just the normal ageing process. And sometimes this may indeed be the case. Even at age eighty five, not everyone has Alzheimer's disease. However, once the symptoms of dementia and possibly Alzheiimer's are diagnosed, the reality must be faced and the issue discussed by all the family.

It is important at this stage, whilst only suffering limited short term memory loss that the patient be part of the process. In fact the patient should make himself as aware of what is happening and might subsequently happen. Even if like myself you believe that you have almost arrested the dementia, you must still be aware of all possible eventualities.

The family participation at this stage is very important, as plans can be made for other family members to learn how to deal with the patient and be able to give the principal caregiver regular breaks. Support for the principal caregiver is critical, as the job may well become more stressful and it is not unknown for otherwise healthy caregivers to die before their patients.

TWENTY NINTH LETTER TO JULIAN

DEMENTIA AND SEXUALITY

Sexual desire does not necessarily change because of dementia. Like the rest of the population many patients remain sexually active, despite ageing and indeed many doctors consider that regular sex is very beneficial to the health.

Sometimes in care homes, relationships between patients do develop, not necessarily sexual in extent, but where there are spouses or partners still at home these can obviously present difficulties. Sadly, in some cases the people themselves do not remember their previous partners and it must be heartbreaking indeed to have been a loving caregiver and now to be forgotten.

This kind of difficulty must be resolved by the care home in an appropriate manner and fortunately such events are rare and modern care homes dealt with in a professional but caring way.

However, inappropriate sexual behavior does sometimes happen. For example touching genitalia, undressing in public, mastabation , and sexual comments or demands. It is of course realized that such behavior is part of the illness and must be dealt with appropriately by gentle discouragement. If this takes place at home, then expert advice must be sought from the local Alzheimer's Care Group, or alternatively from one of the several very helpful Alzheimer sites in the internet.

One of the things to be borne in mind is that everyone needs love and affection. Sometimes this is all that patients are needing .So if possible give hugs and touch your patient in a caring, but appropriate way.

 Exercise can reduce or remove inappropriate sexual behavior. In addition, where speech by the patient has become limited, sometimes the touching of genitalia for example, may indicate that the patient may need to visit the toilet, be changed, or even perhaps be suffering from constipation.

However, with a patient still living at home and in the early to middle stages of dementia the sexual problems may be of a more complex nature. The patient may well still want regular sexual intercourse, but the caregiver may be much less interested. Where the caregiver is the patient's wife or partner, this is perhaps because of the changed dynamic of the relationship. The husband has become much more dependent on the wife, perhaps in some ways almost childlike and thus his status is no longer that of the 'man of the family', but almost that of another child.

From the point of view of the wife or partner desire may fade. This can cause feelings of guilt, but like so many things in the new relationship, there is no simple answer. If you just cannot allow sexual relations to take place, then in the short term you will need to divert attention to something else and hope that the desire of the patient fades, at least for the time being. Talking with a professional counsellor will help to clarify feelings and to deal with the problem. Sometimes increased affection may become a substitute for sexual activity.

Another problem that may develop as the illness progresses, is that the patient may no longer be sexually active, but the caregiver may wish to be so. Bearing in mind that Alzheimer's patients can live for many years, this may become a problem. Frankly there is no simple answer to this dilemma. Much will depend on the caregiver's religious beliefs, but no doubt extra marital relationships do happen. Only the caregiver can judge this situation and only a caregiver can know what it feels like to be in this position. Others should not judge, but human nature being what it is, they will do so. This is especially true of children. Almost everyone who has been divorced and gone into a new relationship will have had to run the gauntlet of 'judgment by offspring.' The question that must be asked is; ' does anyone else need to know'. If not, then your feelings are your own and only you can judge yourself, but do remember that one must always still love oneself.

THIRTIETH LETTER TO JULIAN

RECREATION

From my own experience of looking after someone who was terminally ill I know that boredom can be a big factor. In the case of dementia and Alzheimer's when one's faculties are impaired, but communication is still possible, it is important for both the patient and the caregiver to still have fun. Obviously everyone's idea of fun may be different and there will be limits to the possibilities, but the caregiver must endeavor to create both mental and physical activities if and where possible.

Almost everyone loves going out and to a person whose life has become circumscribed by illness even a visit to McDonalds can be an adventure. Also, it's good for all concerned to keep up social contacts, but people should be as aware as possible of both the fact that any 'odd' behavior is caused by the illness and not the person, but in addition it should be explained that people suffering from Alzheimer's usually retain their intelligence. In fact, in the earlier to middle stages of dementia most of the time the symptoms of Alzheimer's will not be apparent and patients can carry out normal conversations. However, there may be some loss of words and confusion with meanings. In a book I read recently a lady took her elderly father to a restaurant and after perusing the menu he ordered steak and spiders. Although the waiter was to say the least startled, his very quick witted daughter realized that he meant steak and chips. Understanding the Alzheimer language calls for great skill.

Fun at home can be created by encouraging social visits from friends and family and if people are musical a lot of enjoyment can be had from singing, as families did in 'The Old Days.' If someone has, and can play a musical instrument so much the better. Music generally is of course very beneficial to dementia and Alzheimer's patients and should be encouraged and the enjoyment shared if possible. Solitary activities such as reading whilst still possible should be encouraged and painting and model making all help the cognitive abilities.

Apart from activities at home and outside, the patient may be able to enjoy some time at day care centres which are in many cities. If the patient is comfortable meeting other people, then new friends can help to stimulate.

Having fun and relaxing are also of great importance to the caregiver as well as the patient. Plans must be made for this and if the caregiver is going out, or even away for a break this is an excellent idea and no guilt should be felt provided the correct steps have been taken in obtaining and introducing an alternative caregiver.

Depending on the stage of dementia this may have to be done gradually over several visits., so that the patient comes to accept an alternative caregiver. It will need to be done very carefully initially, with the principal caregiver only leaving the room for a few moments and preferably with a brief explanation, such as; "I'm going to make some tea." Or "I must hang out the washing." When deemed appropriate, the caregiver can go for an hour or so to do shopping. Be prepared for the patient to want to accompany and have a diversionary answer ready, such as; "I won't be long." Or "I'm going to bring you back a nice surprise."

Like all things to do with dementia and Alzheimer's thought and planning are required. Truly, the role of the caregiver calls for genius as well as care and love!

THIRTY FIRST LETTER TO JULIAN

ANGER

Whilst a loved one may lose their short term memory and cognitive abilities, it is not always the case that this will be severe. So the caregiving process over the years, should be one of hope that the damage may not get worse. Sometimes deterioration is very slow and so, although being a caregiver is a very laborious activity, both mental and physical, where there has been love it is possible that life can go on in a reasonably comfortable way. Much will depend on individual circumstances.

Very often a patient's behavior will become outlandish and this will be very trying, but by this time the caregiver will hopefully have learnt to divert the patient and how to explain to others discretely the challenges and to gain their understanding and acceptance. Learning to laugh and not to be embarrassed by the odd things that the patient does will help. However, even the patience of a Saint would be tested by the difficulties faced from time to time. The accusations of stealing, infidelity, neglect and so on can sometimes hurt so much that a caregiver's anger will surface and harsh words will result. Of course this should not happen, but it may. If so, the caregiver must take a deep breath and divert the conversation and hopefully both parties will calm down.

Afterwards, it is normal to feel great guilt for having lost ones temper, but caregivers must remind themselves that they are only human and forgive themselves. After all, you do have the hardest job on the planet.

THIRTY SECOND LETTER TO JULIAN

DEATH

When death of a loved one comes, do not feel guilty about how you feel. If death follows a long illness you may feel relief that their suffering is over. You may feel relief that your own constant and attentive labours and attention have come to an end. Do not feel guilt. Rather remember all the attention and love that you have put in to care for your patient and be gentle with yourself.

Talking to another whom you can trust will make your feelings much clearer to yourself. You may well feel loneliness and loss. You may feel as if a great load has been lifted from your shoulders and if so, don't feel guilt.

As I write these words I am conscious of the dilemma of not knowing when you will read them, or if I will be successful over the years to come in containing the dementia and Alzheimer's. I hope that we will have many more years of the great adventure that is life. But whatever comes, know that my wonderful life has been filled with such joy since we met and married that my gratitude to both yourself and God is immense. Truly, I have been so blessed.

Also, after I have gone, know that I will fully understand and accept if you marry again. I will of course still be keeping an eye on you, so look after my dogs and put some flowers from our garden on my grave from time to time!

David

DO NOT ASK ME TO REMEMBER

Do not ask me to remember,

Don't try to make me understand,

Let me rest and know you're with me,

Kiss my cheek and hold my hand

I'm confused beyond your concept

I am sad and sick and lost

All I know is that I need you,

To be with me at all cost,

Do not lose your patience with me,

Do not scold or curse or cry,

Can't help the way I'm acting,

Can't be different though I try,

Just remember that I need you,

That the best of me is gone,

Please don't fail to stand beside me,

Love me till my life is done.

ANONYMOUS

If you love this book, or ate it, or just like it please do feel free to express your feelings.

Apart from my blog barnatod@blogspot.com   I can be contacted by e mail dwheater@lantic.net

Dementia and Alzheimer's are changing in significance all the time. Almost monthly someone claims to have discovered something that will halt or even reverse the two deadly enemies, dementia and Alzheimer's. Unfortunately, when interviewed and asked when their cures will be available they all talk in years. So the numbers of victims grow, but if we can only slow down the advance and liv more comfortably with it, this will be something worthwhile.

Please do feel free to write with stories about yourself or others and ask any questions, all e mails will be replied to.

David.

PICTURE

HOW TO FIGHT DEMENTIA AND WIN

ROUGHLY HALF THE POPULATION AT AGE SIXTY FIVE WILL

HAVE FALLEN VICTIM TO DEMENTIA, WHICH IS THE SYMPTOM

OF DAMAGE TO THE BRAIN AND IN 80% OF VICTIM THE

UNDERLYING DISEASE WILL BE ALZHEIMER,S DISEASE.

ALTHOGH THERE IS AS YET NO KNOWN SCIENTIFIC CURES FOR

DEMENTIA OR ALZHEIMER'S. THERE ARE WAYS TO FGHT THE

DISEASE AND TO SLOW DOWN THE ADVANCE.

DAVID BARNATO HAS HAD DEMENTIA FOR TEN YEARS

AND HAS HAD GREAT SUCCESS IN HOLDING BACK

59

THE ILLNESS AND TO LIVE A VERY HAPPY LIFE. HE

STILL DRIVES A CAR AND HAS WRITTEN THREE NOVELS

AND NOW THIS FASCINATING BOOK ABOUT HOW HE

DEALT WITH THE CHALLENGES AND HOW YOU CAN DO

THE SAME. THE INFORMATION IN THE BOOK INCLUDES

DETAILS OF A NATURAL FOOD THAT HAS HELPRD DAVID

TO ALMOST STOP THE ADVANCE OF DEMENTIA.

DAVID'S WEEKLY BLOG TELLS THE STORY OF HIS CHALLENGES barnatod@blogspot.com

David is 72 and lives with his wife Julian in a small town near Cape Town in South Africa. He can be contacted on

dwheater@lantic.net

www.ingramcontent.com/pod-product-compliance
Lightning Source LLC
Chambersburg PA
CBHW051223170526
45166CB00005B/2019